Low Carb Cookies

20+ Best Low Carb Cookie Recipes

Table of content

Introduction 3

Chapter 1 – Why low carb cookies? Health Benefits of Low Carb Lifestyle 4

Chapter 2 – 8 Recipes of Low Carb Chocolate Chip Cookies 6

Chapter 3 – 7 Recipes of Low Carb Butter, Oatmeals, and Sweetie Cookies 16

Chapter 4 – 8 Recipes of Low Carb Cookies for Christmas and Other Holidays 25

Conclusion 33

Introduction

Low carb cookies are good for weight loss because you can enjoy them as snacks or eat them to satisfy your hunger at the wrong time. In the presence of low carb cookies, there is no need to be bored with the tasteless food that you are forced to eat during your weight loss program. There are numerous recipes that will help you to try delicious low carb cookies to maintain your healthy eating habits. It is proven by various studies that low carb diet can promote faster weight loss. It is a good way to restrict the number of calories because calorie control is the biggest factor to reduce excessive amounts of water and fat from the body.

Health Benefits of Low Carb Cookies

Low carb diet is really popular for many years because it has a number of health benefits. You can reduce weight, prevent cardiovascular disease, cancer, and diabetes. With the help of low carb diet, you can restrict the calorie intake up to 45%. You can enjoy the following health benefits with a low carb diet:

- Reduction in LDL (bad) cholesterol level and reduce your blood pressure
- Increase the HDL (good) cholesterol
- Reduce the risk of type 2 diabetes
- Improve your weight loss rate
- Decrease the risk of cardiovascular disease

This book is particularly designed for you with 23 delicious low carb cookie recipes. These recipes are easy to try and you can make them even with your limited budget. If you want healthy snacks to maintain healthy eating habits, then you should download this book.

Chapter 1 – Why low carb cookies? Health Benefits of Low Carb Lifestyle

If you are fond of cookies then you should avoid high-fat and sugary cookies because these can increase your weight. You can limit the amount of sugar and carbohydrates in cookies with the help of low carb cookies. There are numerous recipes that can help you to bake low-carb cookies with low fat, sugar, and various other healthy ingredients. In low carb recipes, you can reduce the number of ingredients with high carbohydrates, such as flour and sugar. There are different types of low carb cookies that you can try at home, such as low carb butter cookies, oatmeal cookies, chocolate cookies, etc. These are better in taste and shape as compared to regular cookies. In the low carb cookies, you can replace sugar, wheat flour and other similar ingredients that can make you fat.

Benefits of Low Carb Lifestyle

In low carb lifestyle, it is important to reduce the consumption of additional carbohydrates and sugar. A low carb lifestyle will help you to get rid of lots of physical ailments. By adopting a low carb lifestyle, you can enjoy following health benefits:

Reduction in Weight

By following a low carb lifestyle, you will be able to enjoy a good health. It will promote the speed of your weight loss and you can get rid of additional fat easily. It is a successful way to reduce weight because in this way, you completely cut the amount of sugar and take low carbs from your diet.

Improve the Level of Blood Sugar

The low carb diet can reduce the level of fasting glucose and glycated hemoglobin. It is really beneficial for you, particularly for diabetic patients. You can follow this diet to reduce the blood sugar and improve your health.

Reduce High Blood Pressure

High blood pressure is not good for your physical condition because it can amplify the risk of heart attack and stroke. If you want to reduce the blood pressure naturally, then you should follow a low carb diet. It will keep you away from heart diseases and high blood pressure. The obese people should follow this diet to reduce their blood pressure.

Improve Triglycerides in Blood

Fluctuation in the triglyceride level in the blood can be the reason of serious threats. If you want to get rid of these problems and reduce the risk of obesity, diabetes, and other relevant health complications, then you should reduce the level of HDL in the blood. It can be done by reducing the carbohydrates in your diet.

HDL and LDL Cholesterol

The increase in HDL cholesterol can increase the chances of heart diseases; therefore, it is important to restrict carbohydrates in your diet. It will restrict the HDL cholesterol in your blood. LDL is good cholesterol that should be present in your body. It is available in the form of particles, such as fluffy cotton balls. Low carb diet will improve the LDL particle size and you can get rid of coronary heart diseases. With the restriction of carbohydrate, you will have a very good effect on your health. It will improve the particle number of LDL.

Decrease the Level of Insulin Resistance

Insulin resistance is very common in the individuals having metabolic syndrome. It has strong connections with abnormal lipid profile. There would be an association between cardiovascular disease and insulin resistance. Carbohydrate restriction can reduce the insulin resistance and it is better than a low-fat diet.

Reduction in C-reactive Protein

C-reactive protein (CPR) can be calculated in the blood and reduce the chances of inflammation, CRP and heart diseases. It can reduce the chances of various health risks and bring significant improvements in your health.

Chapter 2 – 8 Recipes of Low Carb Chocolate Chip Cookies

If you want to enjoy low carb cookies as snacks with a cup of tea, then there are various variations in recipes that you can try. Try the following recipes of chocolate chip cookies that are easy to bake at home:

Recipe 01: Low Carb Chocolate Chip Cookies

- 1¼ cup flour made of almond
- 3 tablespoons flour (coconut)
- 1 teaspoon vanilla flakes
- ½ teaspoon baking soda
- ¼ cup butter
- ½ teaspoon salt
- 1 egg
- ½ cup sweetener
- ⅓ cup chocolate chips without sugar

Directions:

Prepare the oven at 350 degrees and prepare a baking sheet by placing parchment paper on it. Take a medium sized bowl and sieve almond and coconut flour in it. Pour baking soda and salt into the flour and mix it well. In a separate bowl, whisk cream butter, sweetener, eggs and vanilla to get a smooth mixture. Now add a mixture of flour and baking soda in this mixture and mix them well. Add chocolate chips and mix them properly.

You can use a tablespoon to drop smaller amounts of dough on the baking sheet, but make sure to keep the distance of almost 2 inches between the cookies. Use your hand to make the cookies flat up to desired thickness. Keep the baking sheet in the microwave for almost 10 to 12

Drop 1-2 tablespoon sized heaps of dough onto baking sheets, spacing the mounds at least 2 inches apart. Use the bottom of a clean cup to level the cookies to the preferred size and depth. Bake the cookies for almost 12 minutes and let their edges become golden. Let the cookies cool on the sheet for almost 2 to 3 minutes and then transfer on the wire rack.

Nutritional Information:

Protein 3.71g, Fat 12.24g, Fiber 2.28g, Cals 145, Sugar Alcohols 3.09g, Carbs 7.48g — Total CARBS: 2.11g

Recipe 02: Avocado Chocolate Chip Cookie

- 13 oz Almond Flour
- 1/2 cup brown sugar or sweetener
- 1/2 tsp salt
- 1 egg
- 1/2 tsp baking soda
- 1 stick saline butter
- 1 tablespoon vanilla
- 1/2 cup Chocolate Chips without sugar
- 1/8 cup Water

Directions:

Take a bowl and beat eggs, vanilla, soft butter and mix them well. In another bowl, whisk almond flour, baking soda and salt. Mix the ingredients of both the bowls and add chocolate chips as well. Prepare a baking sheet with parchment paper and pour a small scoop on the sheet. Bake them at 350 degrees in a preheat oven for almost 10 minutes.

Nutritional Information for Each Cookie:

Calories: 119.5, Cholesterol: 16.5 mg, Sodium: 102.0 mg, Total Carbs: 8.1 g, Dietary Fiber: 1.6 g, Total Fat: 11.0 g, Protein: 3.3 g

Recipe 03: Flourless Pumpkin Cookies with Chocolate

- 1/2 cup coconut butter
- 1 egg
- 1/2 cup pumpkin squash
- 1/2 cup stevia
- 2 1/2 teaspoons spice used in pumpkin pie
- 1/4 teaspoon liquid stevia
- 1 teaspoon vanilla extract
- Melted chocolate without sugar

Directions:

Set the temperature of an oven to 350 degrees F, and let it heat. Prepare a baking sheet with parchment paper and keep it aside. Add all ingredients in a food processor to blend them properly. Use a tablespoon to evenly distribute the mixture on the baking sheet with a distance of almost one inch. Place the baking sheet in oven for almost 13 to 15 minutes. Remove from the oven after baking them and let them cool down slightly before sprinkling chocolate.

Nutrition Information for Each Cookie:

Calories: 181, Sugar: 2.7g, Fat: 15.6g, Fiber: 5g, Carbohydrates: 7.7g, Protein: 4.9g, Sodium: 61mg and Cholesterol: 20mg

Recipe 04: Gluten-free Cookies with Chocolate

- 1 teaspoon baking powder
- Vanilla powder or chocolate powder (1 teaspoon)
- 1 1/2 cup flour
- 125 g soft butter without salt
- 1/2 cup rice syrup
- 1 egg
- 1/2 teaspoon sea salt
- 100 g dark chocolate

Directions:

Set the temperature of an oven to 160 degrees C, and let it heat. Prepare a baking sheet with parchment paper and keep it aside. Add all ingredients except chocolate in a food processor to blend them properly. Pour the blend in a bowl and add finely chopped dark chocolate pieces. Use a tablespoon to evenly distribute the mixture on the baking sheet with a distance of almost one inch. Place the baking sheet in oven for almost 15 to 20 minutes. Remove from the oven after baking them and let them cool down slightly before sprinkling chocolate.

Recipe 05: Chocolate Chip Cookies without Egg

- 1 cup and 2 tablespoons all-purpose flour
- ½ teaspoon Baking soda
- Salt (a pinch is enough, but don't use in case of salted butter)
- ½ cup butter without salt
- ¼ cup Granulated sugar and ¼ cup brown sugar
- ½ teaspoon Vanilla extract
- 2 tablespoon milk
- ½ cup Chocolate chips

Directions:

Set the temperature of an oven to 350 degrees F for 10 minutes, and let it heat. Prepare a baking sheet with parchment paper and keep it aside. Add all ingredients except chocolate in a food processor to blend them properly. Use a tablespoon to evenly distribute the mixture on the baking sheet with a distance of almost one inch. Place the baking sheet in oven for almost 13 to 15 minutes. Remove from the oven after baking them and let them cool down slightly before sprinkling chocolate.

Recipe 06: Triple Chocolate Chip Cookies

- 1/2 cup butter without salt
- 1/2 cup brown sugar
- 1/2 teaspoon baking soda
- 1 large egg
- 1/2 teaspoon vanilla flakes
- 1 1/8 cups gluten-free flour
- 1/2 teaspoon salt
- 1 cup chocolate chips (white and brown)

Directions:

Set the temperature of an oven to 375 degrees F, and let it heat. Prepare a baking sheet with parchment paper and keep it aside. Beat butter and brown sugar in a bowl and whisk salt, baking soda and flour in another bowl. Properly beat eggs for 20 to 30 seconds and pour the blends of all bowls in one bowl and add finely chopped dark chocolate pieces. Use a tablespoon to evenly distribute the mixture on the baking sheet with a distance of almost one inch. Place the baking sheet in oven for almost 15 to 20 minutes. Remove from the oven after baking them and let them cool down slightly before sprinkling chocolate.

Nutritional Information of Each Cookie:

182 calories, 9.6 g fat, 22.9 g carbs, 29 mg cholesterol, 128 mg sodium, 2.1 g protein

Recipe 05: Chocolate Chip Cookies without Egg

- 1 1/2 cups furrowed dates
- 1 tablespoon cocoa powder
- 1/8 tsp salt
- A small cup of chocolate chips
- Threadbare coconut
- Melted chocolate

Directions:

Mix dates, cocoa powder, and salt in a strong food processor at a high speed to make a smooth blend. Prepare a mixture in a bowl and make small balls with hands and sprinkle coconut on the cookies. Place the baking sheet in oven for almost 15 to 20 minutes. Remove from the oven after baking them and let them cool down slightly before sprinkling chocolate chips.

Nutritional Information for Each Cookie:

Calories 55, Fat 0.2g, Sodium 20mg, Potassium 141mg, Total carbohydrates 14.7 g

Recipe 07: Cookies of Pecan Coconut Chocolate Chip

- 2 1/2 cups gluten-free flour
- 1 teaspoon baking soda
- 1 cup butter (plain and flavored)
- 1/2 teaspoon salt
- Sweet cream (2 tablespoons)
- 1/2 cup brown sugar
- 2 eggs
- 2 teaspoon coconut + vanilla extract
- 1 1/2 cups coconut flakes
- 1 cup crushed pecans
- 3/4 cup chocolate chips (black and white)

Directions:

Set the temperature of an oven to 350 degrees F, and let it heat. Prepare a baking sheet with parchment paper and keep it aside. Take a bowl and mix butter and brown sugar. In another bowl, you will prepare the mixture of salt, flour and baking soda. Beat eggs and mix coconut extracts and vanilla. Mix all the ingredients in one bowl and blend the mixture well. Use a tablespoon to evenly distribute the mixture on the baking sheet with a distance of almost one inch. Place the baking sheet in oven for almost 13 to 15 minutes. Remove from the oven after baking them and let them cool down slightly before sprinkling chocolate.

Nutrition Information for Each Cookie:

Calories 186, Fat, 11.3, Cholesterol 18, Sodium 103, Sugars 12.4, Dietary Fiber 1, Protein 2.1, Potassium 54, Total carbohydrates 20.1

Recipe 08: Red Velvet Low Carb Cookies

- 15oz Kidney Beans
- 1/2 cup roasted Beet pulp
- 1/4 cup Almond Milk
- 2 tsp coconut flakes
- 2 tsp butter flavor
- 1 tsp Stevia flakes
- 1/4 tsp Salt
- ¾ cup Erythritol 53g
- 2/3 cup Cocoa Powder without sugar
- ¼ cup white flour
- 2 tsp Baking Powder
- 1 tsp White Vinegar

Directions:

In a food processor, process kidney beans, almond milk and extracts to get a smooth blend. Add erythritol and puree as well to get a smooth blend. Set the temperature of an oven to 350 degrees F, and let it heat. Prepare a baking sheet with parchment paper and keep it aside. Mix cocoa powder, flour and bean batter in a bowl to make the batter. Add vinegar to whisk everything to get a smooth texture. Use a tablespoon to evenly distribute the mixture on the baking sheet with a distance of almost one inch. Place the baking sheet in oven for almost 13 to 15 minutes. Remove from the oven after baking them and let them cool down slightly before sprinkling chocolate.

Nutrition Information for Each Cookie:

Total calories 250, Fat 12 g, Sodium 270mg, Sugars 20 g, Total Carbohydrate 25 g, Protein 3 g

Chapter 3 – 7 Recipes of Low Carb Butter, Oatmeals, and Sweetie Cookies

These recipes are perfect for the lovers of butter and oatmeals, then try following recipes in your own kitchen:

Recipe 09: Peanut Butter Cookies with Chocolate

- 1 packet cake mix
- Peanut butter: 1 cup
- Water: 1/3 cup
- 2 eggs
- Peanut butter chips (1 cup)

Directions:

Set the temperature of an oven to 350 degrees F, and let it heat. Prepare a baking sheet with parchment paper and keep it aside. Take a large bowl and mix water, eggs, peanut butter and cake mix. Make a smooth blend and add peanut butter chips. Use a tablespoon to evenly distribute the mixture on the baking sheet with a distance of almost one inch. Place the baking sheet in oven for almost 13 to 15 minutes. Remove from the oven after baking them and let them cool down slightly before sprinkling chocolate.

Nutrition Information for Each Cookie:

Calories 100, Protein 3 g, Carbohydrates 10 g, Fat 5g, Sodium 110 mg

Recipe 10: Applesauce Cookies with Raisin

- Vegetable oil: ¼ cup
- Sugar: ¼ cup
- 1 whole egg
- 1 teaspoon vanilla
- 1/2 cup applesauce without sugar
- 1/2 cup flour (gluten-free)
- 2 tsp powder for baking
- 1/2 tsp baking soda
- 1/2 c flour (unbleached)
- 1 tsp cinnamon
- 1/8 teaspoon clove powder
- 1/2 cup rolled oats
- 1/2 cup raisin

Directions:

Set the temperature of an oven to 375 degrees F, and let it heat. Mix eggs, vanilla, applesauce, oil and sugar in one bowl. Make a blend of cinnamon, oats, baking soda, raisins, flours and remaining ingredients. Prepare a baking sheet with parchment paper. Use a tablespoon to evenly distribute the mixture on the baking sheet with a distance of almost one inch. Place the baking sheet in oven for almost 13 to 15 minutes. Remove from the oven after baking them and let them cool down slightly before sprinkling chocolate.

Nutrition Information for Each Cookie:

Calories 56, Protein 1 g, Carbohydrates 10 g, Fat 2 g

Recipe 11: Special Meringues with Min Chocolate

- 3 eggs (only whites)
- ¼ teaspoon tartar cream
- One pinch salt
- ¾ cup sugar
- 3 tablespoons cocoa
- 1/3 cup chocolate chips
- ¾ teaspoon peppermint flakes
- 5 peppermint candies without sugar

Directions:

Set the temperature of an oven to 250 degrees F, and let it heat. Prepare a baking sheet with parchment paper and keep it aside. Beat egg white and tartar with a mixer and add sugar and cocoa as well. Gently add remaining ingredients and make a smooth blend. Use a tablespoon to evenly distribute the mixture on the baking sheet with a distance of almost one inch. Place the baking sheet in oven for almost 13 to 15 minutes. Remove from the oven after baking them and let them cool down slightly before sprinkling chocolate.

Nutrition Information for Two Cookies:

Calories 70, Total Fat 1.5g, Cholesterol 0 mg, Carbohydrate 15 g, Dietary Fiber 1 g, Protein 1 g, and Sugars 12 g.

Recipe 12: Almond Cookies with Delicious Flavors

- 1/2 cup soft butter
- 3/4 cup sugar
- 1/4 cup egg
- 1/2 teaspoon almond flakes
- 1-1/4 cups flour (all purpose)
- 1/4 teaspoon baking powder
- 1/4 teaspoon powder of cinnamon, cloves, and nutmeg
- A pinch of salt
- 1/2 cup crushed almonds

Directions:

Set the temperature of an oven to 350 degrees F, and let it heat. Prepare a baking sheet with parchment paper and keep it aside. Take a bowl and mix all ingredients one by one to get a smooth blend. Use a tablespoon to evenly distribute the mixture on the baking sheet with a distance of almost one inch. Place the baking sheet in oven for almost 9 to 12 minutes. Remove from the oven after baking them and let them cool down slightly before sprinkling chocolate.

Nutrition Information for Each Cookie:

Calories 85, Fat 4 g, Sodium 62 mg, Carbohydrates 10 g, Fiber 0 g, Protein 1 g

Recipe 13: Macaroons with Cherry and Coconut

- 2 large eggs (whites)
- 1/4 teaspoons tartar cream
- 1/3 cup sugar alternate
- 1 teaspoon almond flakes
- 2 1/4 cups crushed coconut

Directions:

Set the temperature of an oven to 375 degrees F, and let it heat. Prepare a baking sheet with parchment paper and keep it aside. Mix cream, egg white and sugar replacement in a bowl and beat them well. Add almond and coconut extracts in the batter. Use a tablespoon to evenly distribute the mixture on the baking sheet with a distance of almost one inch. Place the baking sheet in oven for almost 20 minutes. Remove from the oven after baking them and let them cool down slightly before sprinkling chocolate.

Nutrition Information for Each Cookie:

Calories 29.2, Fat .851 g, Fiber .275 g, Protein .698 g, Carbohydrates 4.82 g

Recipe 14: Sugar-Free Cookies

- 1/2 cup butter without salt
- 1 cup Granulated sweetener
- 1 tablespoon vanilla
- 1/4 cup egg alternative
- 1/4 cup water
- 3/4 teaspoon vinegar
- 1/4 teaspoon salt
- 1 1/2 cups flour (all purpose)
- 1 1/2 cups flour for cake
- 1 teaspoon powder for baking

Directions:

Set the temperature of an oven to 350 degrees F, and let it heat. Prepare a baking sheet with parchment paper and keep it aside. Prepare the dough with the help of four, butter, vinegar, water and all other ingredients. You can use an electric mixer to blend properly. Divide the dough equally, and cut it with a cookie cutter to place on the baking sheet with a distance of almost one inch. Place the baking sheet in oven for almost 10 to 12 minutes. Remove from the oven after baking them and let them cool down slightly before sprinkling chocolate.

Nutrition Information for Each Cookie:

Calories 60, Fat 3 g, Sodium 30 mg, Total Carbs 7g, Sugars 1 g and Protein 1 g

Recipe 15: Apple and Butter Cookies

- 3/4 cup soft butter
- 1 cup Sweetener
- 2 teaspoons lemon peel
- 2 whole eggs
- 1/2 cup applesauce without sugar
- 1/3 cup apple juice
- 1 3/4 cups flour (all purpose)
- 2/3 cup oats
- 1 teaspoon baking soda
- 1 1/2 teaspoons cinnamon powder
- 1/8 teaspoon nutmeg powder
- 1 cup chopped apples
- 1/2 cup raisins
- 2 teaspoons molasses

Directions:

Set the temperature of an oven to 325 degrees F, and let it heat. Prepare a baking sheet with parchment paper and keep it aside. Prepare the mixture of butter, lemon peel, molasses, the sweetener in a mixture for one minute. Add egg and beat it once again to get a smooth blend. Mix the rest of ingredients one by one and mix them well.

Use a tablespoon to evenly distribute the mixture on the baking sheet with a distance of almost one inch. Place the baking sheet in oven for almost 13 to 15 minutes. Remove from the oven after baking them and let them cool down slightly before sprinkling chocolate.

Nutrition Information for Each Cookie:

Calories 100, Total Fat 5g, Cholesterol 25 mg, Total Carbohydrate 13 g, Sugars 5 g, Protein 2 g, and Dietary Fiber 1g

Recipe 16: Crispy and Delicious Oatmeal Cookies

- 1 1/2 cups oats (old fashioned)
- 1/2 cup flour (all purpose)
- 1/2 cup gluten free flour
- 2 teaspoon cinnamon powder
- 1/2 teaspoon baking soda
- 1/4 teaspoon salt
- 1/3 cup vegetable butter
- 1/2 cup brown sugar
- 1 whole egg
- 1/4 cup raisins
- 1 teaspoon vanilla flakes

Directions:

Set the temperature of an oven to 350 degrees F, and let it heat. Prepare a baking sheet with parchment paper and keep it aside. Mix butter and sugar in a blender. Take another bowl to mix the rest of the ingredients one by one. Make a dough by mixing the contents of both the bowls. Use a tablespoon to evenly distribute the mixture on the baking sheet with a distance of almost one inch. Place the baking sheet in oven for almost 13 to 15 minutes. Remove from the oven after baking them and let them cool down slightly before sprinkling chocolate.

Nutrition Information for Each Cookie:

Calories 98 g, Total Fat 3 g, Total Carbohydrates 17 g, Sugars 8 g, Dietary Fiber 1 g, and Protein 2 g.

Chapter 4 – 8 Recipes of Low Carb Cookies for Christmas and Other Holidays

You can celebrate Christmas and other holidays, without disturbing your diet because followings are some low carb cookies for Christmas and other holidays:

Recipe 17: Gingerbread Cookies

- 1/4 cup soft butter
- 1/4 cup vegetable oil spread
- 1/2 cup sugar (brown)
- 2 teaspoons ginger (powder)
- 1 teaspoon baking soda
- 1 teaspoon cinnamon (powder)
- 1/4 teaspoon cloves (powder)
- 1/4 teaspoon salt
- 1/4 cup molasses (flavored)
- 1 egg
- 2 cups flour (all-purpose)
- 3/4 cup gluten-free flour

Directions:

Set the temperature of an oven to 350 degrees F, and let it heat. Prepare a baking sheet with parchment paper and keep it aside. Take a large bowl and mix butter, vegetable oil spread and beat for almost 30 seconds with an electric mixer. It is time to add ginger, baking soda, salt, cloves, sugar and cinnamon to mix them well. It is time to add flours and mingle to make a dough. Split the dough in half and keep in the refrigerator for almost 2 to 3 hours.

Roll the dough and use a gingerbread cookie cutter to cut out the shapes. Place them on a baking sheet and keep it in the oven for almost 5 to 7 minutes. Remove from the oven after baking them and let them cool down slightly before sprinkling chocolate.

Nutrition Information for Each Cookie:

Calories 73, Fat 2 g, Sodium, 73 mg, Carbohydrates 12 g and Protein 1 gram.

Recipe 18: Almond Cream Star Cookies

- 1/2 cup soft butter
- 1/4 cup cheese (low fat)
- 1 8 ounces almond paste
- 1 teaspoon powder for baking
- 1/4 teaspoon salt
- 1 egg
- 2 1/2 cups flour

Directions:

Take a large mixing bowl, beat the cheese and butter at a medium speed. Add baking powder, almond paste, and salt mix it well. Beat the egg and mix egg and flours in the bowl. Use a wooden spoon to mix the blend and divide the dough in half. Keep it in the refrigerator for almost two hours.

Set the temperature of an oven to 400 degrees F, and let it heat. Prepare a baking sheet with parchment paper and keep it aside. Roll the dough and use a cutter f your desired shape to cut out the cookies and place on the baking sheet with a distance of almost one inch. Place the baking sheet in oven for almost 6 to 8 minutes. Remove from the oven after baking them and let them cool down.

Nutrition Information for Each Cookie:

Calories 66, Total fat 2g, Sodium 40 mg, Carb 7 g

Recipe 19: Butter Cookies with Herbs

- 1/2 cup butter
- 1 egg
- 1 1/2 cups flour (all-purpose)
- 1 cup sugar
- 1 teaspoon powder for baking
- 1/4 teaspoon salt

Directions:

Set the temperature of an oven to 350 degrees F, and let it heat. Prepare a baking sheet with parchment paper and keep it aside.

Beat butter with an electric mixer in a large bowl and add remaining ingredients one by one to blend them well. Divide the dough and make long ropes about 12 inches and keep them in the freezer for 4 hours. Slice the frozen dough and keep on the baking sheet with a distance of almost one inch. Place the baking sheet in oven for almost 13 to 15 minutes. Remove from the oven after baking them and let them cool down.

Nutrition Information for Each Cookie:

Calories 45, Total fat, 1 g, Sodium 33, Carbohydrates 7 g, Protein 1 g

Recipe 20: Delicious Almond Cookies

- Cooking spray
- 2 1/4 cups almonds
- 3/4 cup sugar
- 2 eggs only whites
- 1 teaspoon almond flakes
- Slices of 32 almonds
- 2 ounces melted chocolate

Directions:

Set the temperature of an oven to 350 degrees F, and let it heat. Prepare a baking sheet with parchment paper and keep it aside. Blend all ingredients in a food processor to get a smooth paste.

Use a tablespoon to evenly distribute the mixture on the baking sheet with a distance of almost one inch. Place the baking sheet in oven for almost 13 to 15 minutes. Remove from the oven after baking them and let them cool down.

Nutrition Information for Each Cookie:

Calories 80, Total fat 5 g, Sodium, 4 mg, Carbohydrates 7 g

Recipe 21: Amazing Peanut Butter Cookies

- 1 cup sugar
- 1 cup peanut butter
- 1 egg

Directions:

Set the temperature of an oven to 375 degrees F, and let it heat. Prepare a baking sheet with parchment paper and keep it aside.

Mix peanut butter, egg and sugar in a blender. Use a tablespoon to evenly distribute the mixture on the baking sheet with a distance of almost one inch. Flat-it with your palm or spoon. Place the baking sheet in oven for almost 9 minutes. Remove from the oven after baking them and let them cool down slightly before sprinkling chocolate.

Nutrition Information for Each Cookie:

Calories 66, Total fat 4 g, Sodium 35 mg, Carbohydrates 7 g and Protein 2 g

Recipe 22: Oatmeal Cookies with Fruit

- 2 cups oats (rolled)
- Cooking spray
- 1/2 cup soft butter
- 1 1/2 cups brown sugar
- 3/4 teaspoon soda for baking purpose
- 1/4 teaspoon salt
- 1/4 teaspoon allspice Powder
- 1 6 - ounce low-fat yogurt
- 2 eggs
- 1 teaspoon vanilla
- 2 1/4 cups gluten-free flour
- 1/4 cup crushed walnuts
- 1/4 cup dry apricots
- 1/4 cup dry currants

Directions:

Set the temperature of an oven to 375 degrees F, and let it heat. Prepare a baking sheet with parchment paper and keep it aside.

Take a large bowl and beat butter, now add brown sugar, salt, soda, allspice, yogurt, vanilla and egg to mix everything properly. Mix oats, walnuts, apricots with a wooden spoon and evenly distribute the mixture on the baking sheet with a distance of almost one inch. Place the baking sheet in oven for almost 9 to 12 minutes. Remove from the oven after baking them and let them cool down.

Nutrition Information for Each Cookie:

Calories 101, Total Fat 3 g, Sodium 55 mg, Carbohydrates 17 g, Protein 2 g

Recipe 23: Tasty Thumbprint Cookies

- 6 tablespoons butter
- 1 whole egg
- 1 cup Splenda
- 2 tablespoons milk
- 1 teaspoon vanilla flakes
- 1 1/4 cups gluten-free flour
- 1/4 teaspoon powder for baking purpose
- 1/4 teaspoon baking soda
- ¾ cup fruits of your preference
- 1/4 teaspoon salt

Directions:

Whisk butter, egg, milk and vanilla properly, and now adds flour, salt, baking soda and baking powder. Shape the dough in the form of balls and then place it on a baking sheet.

Set the temperature of an oven to 350 degrees F, and let it heat. Prepare a baking sheet with parchment paper. Shirt the baking sheet in oven for almost 13 to 15 minutes. Remove from the oven after baking them and let them cool down slightly before spreading fruits or unsweetened jam.

Nutrition Information for Each Cookie:

Calories 58, Protein 1 g, Carbohydrates 8 g, Fat 3 g, Cholesterol 16 mg and Sodium 46 mg

Conclusion

If you are incapable of reducing weight, then the use of carbohydrates might be the reason behind it. If you want to reduce a good amount of weight, then you should follow a low carb diet. While following a low carb diet, it is important to consume everything without or with low carbohydrates. The people often make a major mistake while reducing weight that they use normal cookies that are loaded with carbohydrates and sugar.

If you want to increase the speed of your weight loss, then it is important to include low carb cookies in your diet. There are numerous low-carb recipes that are easy to follow and you can try them at home. You can make oatmeal cookies, low sugar cookies, Christmas cookies, peanut butter cookies, etc. You have endless choices, so support your diet plan with the help of low carb cookies.

www.ingramcontent.com/pod-product-compliance
Lightning Source LLC
LaVergne TN
LVHW011559070225
803202LV00010B/782